]

WON'T SLEEP!

The Gentle Fix for Toddlers Who Just Won't Sleep

By Paul Miller

ISBN-13: 978-1540541000
ISBN-10: 1540541002

DEDICATION

Thank you to my wife and best friend, Kristee. Also, in no particular order: Raquel Ann, Steve Scott, Carolina Albano, Alex Pazeto for the cover design, and my editor, Kondria Woods.

INTRODUCTION

Wednesday, 4:42 a.m.

I locked the door and walked out into the night. July in Florida is almost unbearably humid, even in the predawn hours.

So much for getting some exercise.

Leaving the stroller, I strapped Jacob into his car seat and made sure he had his lovey.

My wife and older son were both sleeping soundly, like normal human beings. Not wanting to disturb them, I was off on another nighttime jaunt.

I turned on Stitcher and settled in for two hours of driving and podcasts. At least Starbucks would be open in 20 minutes.

This was getting ridiculous.

●

Like many families, neither one of our kids slept through the night their first year.

A friend of mine once complained that his boy didn't sleep through the night until four months old. It took everything I had not to punch him in the face.

Christopher, our oldest child, didn't sleep a straight eight hours until he was 16 months old.

Jacob was on track to beat Christopher's record. On average, he woke up three or four times a night. Restful nights were a vague memory and a distant hope. Once again, it was time to start sleep training.

But how? What method should we use?

We weren't fans of Cry It Out (CIO), and we'd essentially been trying No Tears without success since Jacob was born.

It was time for a change; something that would actually work.

The Cry It Out method of sleep training just felt cruel. Maybe we were softies. If so, that only extended as far as not wanting him to scream for hours on end. We wanted our sleep, too, without having to get up all the time to rock him back to sleep.

Being realists, we understood that some crying would be involved during sleep training. After all, Jacob was a toddler. It would be another ten to fifteen years before he stopped crying at the drop of a hat. Crying is just a part of life for children.

There had to be a middle ground, something that worked for parents when neither extreme worked.

This short book details what finally worked for us.

My hope is that it will work for you, too.

CHAPTER ONE
SERIOUSLY! WILL HE EVER
SLEEP THROUGH THE NIGHT?!?

Whoever coined the phrase "sleep like a baby" should be dragged into the street and shot at high noon.

A Family Affair

Our first son, Christopher, taught my wife, Kristee, and me, the *real* meaning of that phrase by waiting until he was a year-and-a-half old before sleeping through the night.

It seemed that no sooner had our oldest finally gotten the hang of sleeping then our second was born.

Back to thrice-midnight feedings and sleepless nights. Like the return of a chronic migraine, it's familiar, but not a friend. Like his brother before him, Jacob couldn't figure out how to sleep through the night on his own.

We've had maybe one year of peaceful sleep out of the last four, and we count ourselves lucky.

Jacob, our youngest, was 16 months old when we knew it was time. Although he had weaned himself from breastfeeding at nine months, he still relied on the bottle and rocking chair to fall asleep.

We knew this was a possibility even before he was born. While everyone tells you that every child is different, we were somewhat pessimistic and assumed some of the negatives, such as sleepless nights, would be the same.

We were right.

While we were prepared, it was still exhausting.

My wife took the brunt of the burden. A stay-at-home mom, she felt the need to let me sleep so I could be rested for work. While I took a small share of the nights, the effort she put forth was incredible. To average four hours of chronically interrupted sleep and still raise two boys was incredible to witness.

But there comes a time when enough is enough. We're not meant to live on such a minimal amount of sleep. It takes physical, mental, and emotional tolls, even on the best of us.

We were also worried that the boys wouldn't be able to share a bedroom for years to come. Blessed to have a three-bedroom home, Christopher and Jacob each had their own rooms. We didn't think it'd be fair to Christopher to put Jacob in the same room, only to have both of them wake up several times throughout the night.

Doing Everything Right… and Failing

At sixteen months, Jacob had only slept through the night once.

We thought we'd done everything right. Our responses to crying were consistent: we always picked him up and rocked him back to sleep.

Believing the saying "sleep begets sleep," we'd let him nap as long as possible. That just meant he'd stay up until 9:30 at night, well past the time we felt he should be in bed.

We tried limiting his naps and keeping him up until he was practically asleep on his feet.

We never co-slept. While we did keep him in a cradle in our room for the first few months, we moved him to his own room when he was four months old.

We adhered to a consistent bedtime of 8:00 p.m. as often as possible. An hour before bed, we eliminated as many sources of stimulation as possible by turning off computer screens, silencing music, and dimming the lights.

Our response to midnight crying was consistent: we made sure his white noise machine was still playing, picked him up, patted and shushed him, and put him back in his crib after he fell back asleep.

We tried stuffing him full of food before bedtime. Honestly, this wasn't too difficult. Jacob showed an early interest in solids, and was still in the phase where he usually liked to try new foods. We'd actually stopped feeding him bottles outside of the bedtime and midnight hours.

Jacob would often run to the kitchen and try opening the pantry an hour after dinner, and get mad when we wouldn't give in. Rather than feeding him the sugary pouches he could grab on his own, we would try slightly less sugary snacks such as graham crackers and Ritz crackers.

When that didn't help, our chiropractor suggested healthy fats such as almond butter and coconut oil. He'd eat two or three tablespoons of almond butter before signing that he was all done.

He still woke up in the middle of the night.

We were at our wit's end. It was time to teach him how to sleep, but we weren't sure how to do it.

What's Normal, Anyway?

What's the deal? Why is it that infants can fall asleep so easily, while babies and toddlers have a harder time? Why can't they sleep through the night like everyone else?

Is this even normal?

Well, kind of.

Researchers at the University of Canterbury in New Zealand published a study about babies and sleep in 2010. They found that more than 50% of babies have "normal" sleep patterns, which were defined as (1) sleeping from midnight to 5 a.m., (2) 10 p.m. to 6 a.m., or (3) any uninterrupted eight-hour stretch. The ability to adhere to these sleep patterns was called "sleep regulation."[1] Of course, that means that almost 50% of babies *don't* have sleep regulation.

It seems that sleepless babies aren't anything to worry about.

But what about older babies and toddlers?

That's where things start to change. As babies mature, the majority of them develop sleep regulation.

In fact, the Canterbury researchers reported that 73% of one-year-olds slept between 10:00 p.m. and 6:00 a.m. Of those, 86% slept for *more* than eight hours a night!

In other words, toddlers like ours who *don't* sleep through the night are actually in the minority.

Welcome to the club! Tell me... how do I upgrade to Platinum level?

So, why do some children struggle with sleeping through the night? It turns out that it's perfectly normal, albeit a little less common in toddlers.

According to research reviewed by Dr. Andrew Guthrie from Oklahoma University, this seeming inability to sleep through the night is probably related to something called Developmental Separation Anxiety, or DSA.[2]

Between 10 and 12 months of age, babies experience this normal part of their development.[3] It's likely a result of "object permanence," which is their newfound ability to remember something — or someone — after it leaves their sight.

You probably remember when this started happening. Before the development of object permanence, you could remove a toy from your baby's field of vision and he would forget about it. Ditto for when you left the room.

It's kind of like the notion of hiding under a blanket to escape the monsters. If they can't see you, you must not be there.

After object permanence sets in for your child, they *know* when you've left the room. And because children rely on us for everything, they get worried when we leave. While understandable, it's still frustrating when you feel like you can't even have 30 seconds of privacy in the bathroom!

DSA typically subsides by the time children reach their second birthday,[3] as they start to explore and exert some control over their worlds.

Viewed through the context of DSA, your child's inability to fall asleep by themselves makes sense.

If they're accustomed to falling asleep with a bottle, that means they associate sleep with two things: first, a bottle, and second, you feeding them. If you're anything like us, you probably feed them, then burp and/or gently bounce them until they're asleep.

Then, as a pharmacist friend of mine once described it, you very carefully set them down, just like a live grenade, afraid that one wrong move will result in a devastating explosion.

The problem is your fear of the explosion actually makes it *more* likely to happen. You've trained them in a particular routine.

What happens when you put them down while they're still awake, even just groggy after a feeding?

The second you walk away, two things happen: first, the routine has changed, and that makes your child nervous. Second, DSA kicks in.

RED ALERT! MOMMY'S LEAVING ME!

Cue the explosion.

This same principle explains why your toddler can't go back to sleep after waking up in the middle of the night.

DSA strikes again. What has happened is that your child's environment has changed since they fell asleep. Remember, you were there, feeding and rocking them until they drifted off to sleep. When your child wakes up at midnight (or like ours did at 11 p.m., 12:30 a.m., 2:15 a.m., 3:45 a.m....) and discover you've vanished, they freak out.

How Much Sleep Does Your Toddler Really Need?

Like so many other things about human development, the answer is "it depends."

There's no scientific standard for how much sleep your child actually needs.[4] Those charts you see in all the parenting magazines? They're based on *reported* sleep.

For example, if researchers studied 30 14-month-olds and found that 10 slept for an average of six hours, 10 for an average of seven hours, and 10 for an average of 12 hours, they would report that the average sleep duration was 8.3 hours.

It makes sense if you think about it. Scientists aren't going to deliberately wake kids up early on a consistent basis just to see how bad it is for them! Likewise, they can't force kids to sleep longer than they want to... just as we, parents, can't either, even when we want to.

So, we evaluate our children against the averages. This works as a general rule, but neglects the outliers. After all, an average is only useful when describing the majority. When it comes to human behavior, there are almost always small groups at either end of the spectrum.

Four researchers from the University Children's Hospital in Switzerland were curious about how much sleep children averaged at various stages of development. They studied 493 children, beginning at just one month of age and continuing until they were 16 years old.

They discovered that newborns actually slept anywhere from nine to 19 hours a day![5] If

you were to simply take the average —
14 hours — and assume it was a rule *instead of*
just an average, you might be worried if your
otherwise happy, healthy newborn was only
sleeping 12 hours instead of 14. On the flip
side, you might also worry if they slept *19* hours
a day... but probably not as much.

The amount of sleep the human body
requires is probably determined by growth rate,
exposure to disease, and other conditions.
There's probably a genetic component, as well.[6]
It varies by culture, too: Chinese and Italian
babies get less sleep than their counterparts in
America and the Netherlands.[7,8,9]

So, what's a parent to do?

Trust yourself. As a parent, you probably
have a pretty good idea of how much sleep
your toddler needs. You know that if they only
get 10 hours of sleep during a 24-hour period
when their average is 14 hours, then disaster
threatens. You've seen it first-hand: moodiness,
irritability, and a lack of energy.

When all else fails, trust your instinct.

It's Important for YOU

Let's not forget about ourselves. Becoming an
adult doesn't change the fact that we still need

sleep. As with children, the amount you need depends on health, stress, and perhaps genetics.

And, just as with children, insufficient sleep causes problems such as anxiety, crankiness, and a lack of energy. The other challenge is emotional. The longer you go without regular sleep, the harder it is not to point the finger at your child.

I mean, it's not like you'd intentionally set your alarm to wake yourself at random times throughout the night. It *is* a result of having children. It can be tempting to start to resent them for taking over this part of your life. While it's not their fault, it is because of them.

There's nothing wrong with regretting the fact that you're not well-rested. While it might not be politically correct to talk about, it *is* normal to actually feel some resentment towards your children when you're chronically tired. Just be mindful of your attitude, and recognize that "this too shall pass."

With that out of the way, let's fix the problem and get ready for a new normal!

CHAPTER TWO
THE ELUSIVE ANSWER

The Majority Isn't Always Right

Your search for answers probably followed a similar path to ours. After realizing that our son wasn't going to sleep through the night on his own, we searched online: Google, Amazon, and a Facebook mom's group.

As you might expect, we found two main solutions: Cry It Out and No Tears.

Cry It Out

The basic principle of the Cry It Out (CIO) approach is one of habit change. Children who can't fall asleep on their own, either at bedtime or after a nighttime waking, have learned to depend on their parents to be nursed or rocked to sleep. That habit needs to be changed so your child can learn how to go to sleep by himself.

The two most popular methods of the CIO approach are the Weissbluth Method and the Ferber method.

The primary Weissbluth method is referred to as "extinction." After making sure that your child is napping regularly and that multiple family members help with the bedtime routine, the parent puts their child to bed while drowsy. While you monitor the child from another room to ensure they're safe, you don't return... no matter how long they cry.

Dr. Marc Weissbluth writes that it takes just one to three nights for the child to learn how to sleep on their own.

We tried this *once* with Christopher. After 25 minutes of feeling like horrible parents, we picked him up and vowed never to do it again.

Ferber advocates placing your child down while he's drowsy, returning to check in and comfort him if he starts crying. The time between check-ins gradually increases, from three minutes to 10 the first night, and longer intervals as the days go by. The theory is that your child will eventually learn how to fall asleep without being fed or rocked to sleep.

This works well for many children. For others, though, it can quite literally take *hours* before they fall asleep, exhausted from crying for so long.

Is Cry It Out actually harmful to your child? Experts still don't agree. In a 2011 article for *Psychology Today*, Dr. Darcia Narvaez made the case that CIO actually *decreases* a child's independence and might make them more anxious and uncooperative later in life.[10]

Doctors William and Martha Sears, who answer parenting questions at AskDrSears.com and have raised eight children themselves, do not recommend a Cry It Out approach to sleep training. Being chronically unresponsive to a baby or toddler who is crying does nothing to build parent-child trust.[11]

On the flip side, a 2012 study by Dr. Anna Price from the Centre for Community Child Health and her peers found no long-term emotional or mental harm.[12]

Regardless, we decided that CIO isn't appropriate for our family. Our decision was based on our instincts and our experience from trying it for a short period of time.

No Tears

The belief behind the No Tears method is that leaving your child to cry himself to sleep can cause emotional trauma, both for baby and for mom and dad.

In her book, "The No-Cry Sleep Solution," Elizabeth Pantley tells parents to use their normal routine for placing their children to sleep (or back to sleep), and suggests that they shorten the duration of rocking, shushing, etc., until the child learns how to sleep.

Pantley urges parents to make sure their child is eating enough, has a consistent bedtime routine, and is comfortable in bed. These are critical for setting your child up for restful nights.

While the No Tears method works for many families, we worried that it would prove too exhausting to be sustainable for however long it would take for Jacob to learn how to sleep on his own. We needed our sleep, and Jacob needed to learn this lesson for himself.

Would he figure it out eventually? Of course. But we wondered how long would that take? Another month? Six months? A year?

On the Right Track

Wanting another way, we turned to a family friend, Raquel, who works as a doula. She has gone through this with many children, and we wanted to leverage her advice. After talking with her at length about our experiences and our frustration, we changed how we approached sleep with Jacob.

As soon as he was done with his bottle, we burped him for a few seconds, then placed him down while he was still awake. Of course, he stood right back up.

Raquel's guidance was to lay him back down if he was standing *and* crying. Standing silently was fine, as was lying down and crying. We figured he probably wouldn't stay lying down while crying, so we weren't too worried about that.

We laid him back down and tucked him in, then stepped out of the room.

Through his closed door, we could hear him stand back up as he cried. What followed was a cycle where we returned to his room if he was standing and crying, laid him back down and tucked him in, then we left. If he was standing quietly or crying while lying down, we would leave him alone. This continued for about 40 minutes, until he finally fell asleep.

Kristee and I had just tried an approach that would work for our family. We'll go into detail in the next chapter.

CHAPTER THREE
THE GENTLE SOLUTION

A Method for the Rest of Us

Let's start with a word of warning: if you're the kind of parent who refuses to accept even a second of crying, this method is not for you. While we rejected the Cry It Out approach, we were realistic. Jacob was a young toddler. It would be foolish to approach every learning opportunity with the belief that no crying should occur. News flash: kids cry. It's normal. They cry from the day they're born, up until... oh, I don't know, age 13... or older?

The good news: *excessive* crying has no place in our method.

The Method

- Keep a consistent routine.
- Place your toddler down while he's still groggy. Most toddlers prefer to start on their sides.

- Tuck him in, briefly rub his back (just a few gentle circular motions).

- Leave the room.

- If he starts crying, figure out if he's standing or still lying down.

  o A baby monitor with a camera feature or an independent video camera is a great help to determine this.

  o Otherwise, stand outside his door - you should be able to hear a difference, whether it's his moving to a standing position, or a change in the volume or origin of his crying.

- If he's standing, lay him back down, tuck him back in, and briefly rub his back.

- No talking and no eye contact! Make gentle shushing sounds until he stops crying.

- Step out of the room.

- If he stands up and cries again, go back, lay him down, tuck him back in, and soothe him. Again, don't leave until he stops crying.

HELP! MY TODDLER WON'T SLEEP!

- Repeat until he stops getting up.

Special Situations

What if He Cries While Still Lying Down?

That's okay, unless he's hysterical (or, of course, in pain). If he is, it is perfectly acceptable to return to his side. But *don't* pick him up. If he uses them, make sure he still has his pacifier and lovey. Tuck him back in. Rub his back and maybe his head, and soothe him with gentle shushing sounds.

If he starts crying again as soon as you make a move for the door, use your judgment. Is his crying at a more normal volume, or even whimpering? If so, go ahead and step out. But if he's starting to escalate again, return to his side and repeat the comforting process.

In some situations, you might be able to calm him simply by staying in the room. Leave the lights off, but just sit somewhere where he can see or sense you. We did this on a few occasions and it was a great way to let him know that we were still close, but that it was time to go to sleep.

On one particularly rough occasion, Jacob woke up at 12:55 a.m. and wouldn't go back down. At 1:30 a.m., after a few cycles of laying him down and him sitting right back up, I lay down on the guest bed, adjacent to his crib. Just being physically in the same room seemed to help.

He let out two short cries during that time, both of which I was able to calm simply with a few seconds of shushing from my bed. He finally fell asleep at 2:45 a.m.

What if He's Standing But Not Crying?

That's okay. It's entirely possible that he does that while you're sleeping, and you never knew until you watched him on camera.

If he starts crying, then of course return and repeat the process. If he falls asleep standing up, you may choose to go in and gently lay him back down. Be prepared for him to wake up when you do this, but understand that he'll probably fall back asleep fairly quickly.

Bedtime Routines

If you have a routine, don't change it during sleep training. Disruptions to routines are often hard for toddlers, especially at bedtime. For us, that meant a routine that averaged around 30 minutes. But if your routine is longer, that's okay. Although we don't give our kids baths right before bed, many parents do. There's a lot of anecdotal evidence that a bath before bedtime helps kids relax and unwind in preparation for bed.

With both kids, we made the decision early on to avoid overly-complex, drawn out bedtime routines. The last thing we wanted to do was introduce too many variables. The greater the number of variables, the greater the chance for an unplanned disruption.

In retrospect, maybe that's where we went wrong.

Oh well, no real harm done: both boys *love* baths. These are playful times that are almost viewed as treats for them.

At any rate, our routines are fairly simple. For Jacob, that means a last change of the night, followed by low lighting, no screen time and, when he wants it — which is most of the time — being held.

You'll find a step-by-step schedule of our youngest child's bedtime routine below. I listed some times as ranges, since there's a little variation in actual time, depending on how our night has progressed. Again, your routine and your bedtime may vary. That's okay, just stay consistent!

1. Around 7:15 p.m.: Change into nighttime diaper. Generally, around this

time he wants to be held more than earlier, so I can tell he's getting tired.

2. Between 7:30 p.m. and 7:45 p.m.: Change into pajamas. By this time, I've usually been holding him quite a lot. Bedtime is near. If he doesn't already have them, we'll give Jacob his pacifier and lovey.

3. 8:00 p.m.: Heat up a bottle of milk. One of us will take him upstairs to his room, turn on white noise and ensure that it's set to repeat, turn off the light, and close the door most of the way. We do leave the door cracked, and I'll tell you why in just a minute. We'll feed him while sitting in the rocking chair.

4. 8:05 p.m.: After about 5 minutes, he's usually done. More often than not, he'll finish the bottle. We then stand up, burp him for about 15 seconds, then lay him down in his crib. I'll make sure he's on his side, tuck him in, and rub his back a few times.

Now, here's how we were able to teach him to go to sleep on his own:

1. I'll straighten up and quietly back away from his crib. If he's not moving, I'll ease out of the room through the door. If I left it cracked far enough when I came in, I don't need to open it further to leave. This is important, as he started to associate the opening door with us leaving. Remember: leaving makes children anxious.

2. If he sits back up and starts crying, I'll immediately return and gently lay him back down on his side. I'll tuck him back in and rub his back, which is usually enough to have him stop crying. We found that this happened most often when we closed the door behind us in step 1. Once we started leaving it open, the crying episodes dramatically decreased. This is likely because he knows we're still there, and has probably associated a closed door with separation.

   It's perfectly normal for your toddler to stand right back up and start crying the first time you do this. That's to be expected, as this is a new routine. Show him that you're still there by immediately returning, laying him back down, then soothing him (remember to soothe him after laying him back down, not before!). We had to repeat this cycle for an hour one night, but we knew he was adjusting. Don't be surprised if it takes about a week for your child to adjust to this new routine. But don't quit, either... you'll just confuse him, and make your next try that much harder on both of you. Trust me.

3. Once he's asleep, we'll quietly close the door. While it's helpful to have a camera with night vision in the room, it's certainly not essential. You've probably become hypersensitive to what each of your toddler's sounds mean, and can tell with an ear to the door if he's lying down, sitting, or standing.

The biggest change we made was not rocking him to sleep. The techniques I shared above are what we used to ease his transition from being fully dependent on us – where we put him to bed only after he was asleep – to learning how to go to bed while still awake. By showing him that he's not truly alone, we've found a way to ease the natural separation anxiety he has previously experienced.

While we always try to put him down groggy, it's not always possible. If he falls asleep with the bottle or during the 15 seconds of burping, no harm done. We certainly don't wake him back up just to put him down tired!

Light at the End of the Tunnel

The method I described in this chapter worked for us when it seemed like nothing else would. How long did it take? It sounds almost cliché, but we started seeing results almost immediately. From Day 2, Jacob actually slept through the night four nights in a row. The second week, he slept through the night four out of seven nights, averaging one nighttime waking for each of the remaining three nights. That was significantly better than the three to four nighttime wakings he was averaging before we started. As time went on, his average "compliance ratio" — the percentage of nights he slept straight through without a nighttime waking — continued to improve.

Naps were a little more challenging. The first week was rough. The second week was dominated by so many doctor's appointments and errands that he started most of his naps in the car.

That said, the habits we were building at night seemed to have a good carryover. I remember one Sunday in particular towards the end of our third week. Kristee put Jacob down for a nap just after 2:00 in the afternoon. At 3, he stood up and started crying. By the time I walked into his room, he was already calming down. I laid him down, tucked him back in, and left. He fell back asleep almost immediately, and stayed down for another 45 minutes. An hour and 45 minutes was a great afternoon nap for him, so we considered that a success.

Don't get discouraged when (not if!) you experience ups and downs. You may have nights where it takes an hour to put your toddler to sleep, or two hours to put him back to sleep after a midnight waking. We had several nights like that, and they weren't fun. Fortunately, those should be exceptions, not the norm.

Keep a written log of your sleep training and use it as your reference. Take heart if you see improvement as the days and first two weeks go by.

If you don't see improvement after three weeks, customize the method, or ditch it for something else. As my wife and I can attest, no one method works for everyone. That's bound to be true for ours, as well. If you don't see improvement no matter what method you try — provided you're not bouncing from one to another without giving each one a solid three-to-four weeks — it may be best to consult your pediatrician or a sleep consultant.

Sample Schedule

Here's a sample bedtime schedule, based on the routine that worked for us:

5:30 p.m. - 6:15 p.m.: Dinner.

6:30 p.m. - 7:15 p.m.: Active Play.

7:15 p.m. - 7:30 p.m.: Quieter Play. No screens or noisy toys. Change Pandora from upbeat music to something a bit more calm.

7:30 p.m.: Feed almond butter or other filling, higher fat/low sugar snack (optional).

7:30 p.m. - 7:45 p.m.: Change into nighttime diaper and pajamas.

7:45 p.m. - 8:00 p m.: Offer to hold your baby as much as he wants. Some young toddlers enjoy light massages of their backs and heads as you walk around with them. This can relax and calm them.

8:00 p.m.: Give them a night-time bottle in their room with the lights off. If you plan on weaning your child from the bottle, *do not do so* until *after* they have learned how to go to sleep without help and have consistently done so for several weeks. Of course, if they self-wean, don't force it on them!

CHAPTER FOUR
HOW TO HANDLE
HABITUAL WAKINGS

Sunday, 2:21 a.m.

At least the guest bed was comfortable.

It started during the witching hour. Jacob had been awake since 12:56 a.m., and I was pretty sure I'd finally worn him down. Just before 1 a.m., I laid Jacob down and tucked him in, only to have him sit back up and start crying. This cycle repeated itself five times.

Eventually, I started leaving the bedroom door cracked open about a quarter of the way after leaving. I'm guessing he assumed I was still nearby since he hadn't seen the now-familiar pattern of the door closing. He stayed down, but still let out several loud cries. One of his canine teeth had been poking through his gums for awhile, taking its sweet time to grow out. Figuring that was the source of some pain, I gave him some medicine at 1:45 a.m.

Then, I finally wised up. I lay down in the guest bed in his room and just relaxed as he rolled around in his crib. He seemed to take comfort just from my being there. He let out two pretty good cries, but I calmed him right back down without getting up, just by making shushing sounds. He finally fell asleep after 90 minutes.

Something similar had happened later in the week, on Thursday, when he was awake from 1 a.m. until about 2:45 a.m. That was the first night we tried leaving the door cracked open fairly wide after we left, only closing it after he'd finally fallen asleep.

Stop Wasting Gas at 3 a.m.

Fortunately, those two+ hours of midnight wakings were the exception, not the norm. That said, midnight wakings won't disappear overnight.

Your toddler will probably still wake up during the night. You taught them that it was okay to go to sleep without you, but they still expect you to be there when they wake up.

The strategy for dealing with midnight wakings is essentially the same as the bedtime strategy. If you're still allowing midnight feedings, stop! Aside from separation anxiety, this is one of the main reasons they wake up at night. They're used to being fed!

After we got back from a trip, and before we began sleep training, we eliminated midnight bottles. Instead held or rocked him back to sleep. Once we started sleep training, we followed the steps below for midnight wakings.

1. Walk in and close the door about half-way. Give him his pacifier and lovey, if he's lost either one of them. Lay him down on his side and start shushing him. Tuck him in and rub his back and/or head, continuing to shush him until he stops crying.

2. Start backing away. If he stands up and starts crying again, immediately return and gently lay him back down on his side. Tuck him in and rub his back a few times, then back away again. This cycle was repeated until he stayed down.

   Remember, it's probably going to take some time for your toddler to adjust. Our hardest midnight adjustment started early one Thursday morning. We were one week into sleep training, and it had gone remarkably well. However, for some reason, this night was different. Jacob woke up at 1 a.m. and kept getting back up. At 2:30 a.m., my wife woke me up for the hand-off so she could go back to bed. I definitely got the better end of that bargain, as it was only another 11 minutes before he fell asleep. On that occasion, we made a minor adjustment: easing out hadn't been working, so instead of leaving, I just sat down on the guest bed in Jacob's room. He stayed down but cried for another minute. Then he quieted and, after another few minutes, he stood up. I put him right back down, rubbing his back as usual. He stayed down and drifted off to sleep.

Again, it's helpful to have a camera, but not essential. If your child stands back up but doesn't cry, that's okay. You can choose to lay him back down if you want to, but we didn't generally find that necessary, except on one occasion where Jacob fell asleep standing up with an arm over the edge of his crib!

3. Once he's asleep, we'll quietly close the door and go back to bed.

It may take your toddler several days or even a few weeks to adjust to this new normal. Be persistent, though, because the end result is worth it.

You may have to make adjustments as you go along. While we left the door cracked for a week during sleep training, we started finding that it actually prevented him from going back to sleep. During our third week of sleep training, we kept the door almost completely closed so he wouldn't see ambient light from the hallway outside his room.

By the way, if your child sits up, that is fine. If he's quiet, you might not even notice. We didn't always have cameras in our boys' rooms. In fact, we didn't put a camera in Christopher's room until he was 10 months old. The first time we saw him sitting up quietly an hour or two after bedtime, we rushed in and rocked him back to sleep. It wasn't until the fourth or fifth night of this that we realized it probably wasn't anything new. Who could say that he wasn't sitting up in bed *before* we got the camera, eventually falling back asleep on his own?

If they're sitting and crying, use your best judgment. We did not go in and calm him until he stood up and cried, *unless* he was in hysterics.

A Bit of Advice

Whenever you're starting a new habit, whether it's for yourself or for your children, remember that consistency is key. The old saying that habits take 21 days to form exists for a reason. Think about it: if you want to start working out, you have to do so consistently. Following a haphazard schedule and skipping workouts is virtually guaranteed to result in a cancelled gym membership. The same applies to sticking to a diet, taking up running, potty training your child, etc.

Be fair to yourself and your toddler. Once you start sleep training, commit to following through. Quitting half-way through the process will frustrate you and your toddler, and make it that much harder the next time you try.

Create a plan ahead of time for your toddler's sleep (and waking) schedule, as well as your responses to hysterics, teething, sickness, and other special situations. Remember, be reasonable! If your toddler's bedtime is 8:00 p.m., but he can't keep his eyes open at 7:15 p.m., put him to bed. The longer you wait, the crabbier he'll get... and, paradoxically, the more likely he'll be to wake up during the night.

Do *not* co-sleep, no matter what you used to do. That's a *huge* crutch your toddler doesn't need. Remember, the point of sleep training is to teach your toddler that he can go to sleep without your constant touch. Co-sleeping at any point during training, no matter how challenging the night, will just confuse him more.

Now, use some common sense. If he's in pain, pick him up and figure out the problem. You don't need me to tell you that your toddler's safety should always be your primary concern!

Don't cave in and take him for a car ride, either. You'll just reinforce your child's belief that he is only capable of napping in the car. Learn from our mistakes!

Stick to your plan and you will make it through this.

CHAPTER FIVE
YOUR PINT-SIZED ALARM CLOCK

Sunday, 5:30 a.m.

"It's 5:30. Why is he crying in his crib?"

I was just about to head back up to Jacob's room when my wife poked her head out of the stairwell, bleary-eyed. The cycle of crying-silence-crying-silence had driven her out of bed.

"Uh... because it's 5:30 in the morning?"

Jacob had just slept for nine hours straight, the third night in a row. I was trying to get him to sleep until 7.

"I thought," she replied patiently, "that we had agreed he could get up when one of us was up for the day."

Plan Your Wake-Up Time

She was right, as usual. I tend to forget some of these details, and often set goals that are a bit too farfetched.

Sleep training takes time. When it comes to toddlers, it's important to remember that you're working to change a habit that's been with them their entire lives. Be patient and concentrate on progress, not the ultimate goal.

My advice to you is to agree with your partner on a wake-up time *before* you start sleep training. It's much easier to establish your guardrails going into sleep training, rather than forcing a discussion in the early morning hours while your toddler cries in the background.

Every family and situation is different. What worked for us may work for you, or may sound like insanity. Whether or not you follow our path, the important thing is to set and agree to some guidelines first.

Here's what worked for us. We decided that Jacob could get up at whatever a normal wake-up time was for us. Since my alarm goes off at 4:45 a.m., in theory Jacob could get up then as well. I know that sounds crazy, but in all actuality, it worked pretty well. And yes, I accepted the fact that he could get up as early as 4:45 on the weekends, as well. You might be thinking, *Did he actually wake up around 5 in the morning?* A few times, sure. But they tended to be the exception, rather than the rule.

We also started training him to recognize the difference between midnight and morning. When it was time to wake up for the day, we'd walk in, turn his white noise machine off, and exclaim, "Good morning!" Although I have no scientific basis for it, I believe this helped him get through midnight wakings a bit more easily.

Even on the weekends, I prefer an early riser over one that wakes up crying three times a night! I knew the time would come that he would start waking up later. After all, we don't always wake up at the same time without an alarm clock, do we? Our four-year-old certainly doesn't. While he's fairly consistent, it's usually within the later end of a time frame from 6:45 a.m. to 7:45 a.m.

So, don't worry. While every toddler is different, your early riser just might learn to sleep a little later as his new bedtime and midnight routine solidifies.

And if he wakes up an hour before the scheduled time? Treat it like a midnight waking.

CHAPTER SIX
NAP TIME STRATEGIES

Consistency is Key

Nap time sleep training won't differ too much from bedtime training, except in a few common-sense areas.

As with bedtime, commit to keeping a consistent schedule and routine as much as possible. If your toddler's typical nap times are 10:00 a.m. and 2:00 p.m., for example, try not to deviate too much from those times.

Of course, life gets in the way. You'll probably have doctor's appointments and a day or two full of essential errands. That's normal. While you should do what you can to schedule around naps, sometimes that's just not realistic. Do your best.

Sometimes, your toddler may fall asleep in the car. If you've got some time, keep driving around until he wakes up. If you have to get him out of the car early, you'll naturally try to keep him asleep as you walk into the store.

When you're at home, the important thing is to help your child learn that he can nap without you. Feed him, if that's part of your routine, burp him, and lay him down groggy, just like bedtime. If he sits up, lay him back down.

Exceptions (Reality Check)

Sometimes, your toddler is freaking out and you can tell the looming nap isn't going to happen without extraordinary intervention. If this happens, it's okay to push nap time back *if* you haven't already tried to put him down. Once you start the bedtime routine, you should not stop.

The same thing applies to accidental early wakings, but again, as an exception.

One Sunday morning, Jacob napped from 10:30 a.m. until noon. When I went to his room, he seemed very alert, as if nap time was done. An unsuspecting victim, I turned off his white noise CD, said "Good morning," picked him up, and headed downstairs.

Less than 90 seconds later, during the process of changing his diaper, he flipped. He was kicking, screaming, and trying to shred his lovey with his teeth. As experienced parents, we could tell that he *wasn't* done with his nap, after all!

However, it was too late to take him back to bed. Doing so would just confuse him... and probably give him an opportunity to bash a hole in the wall!

So, I took him for a car ride. In less than two minutes, he fell asleep... and slept another two hours!

The point here is that you have to be prepared to manage exceptions. Just try to minimize them.

CHAPTER SEVEN
CLOSING THOUGHTS

Sleep training takes time and patience. It took us about three weeks before the habits truly solidified for Jacob. He seemed to get comfortable with being placed down groggy towards the end of the first week. On average, his nighttime wakings dropped from three to one the first week. Your mileage may vary. It may be faster for you, or it may take longer. Here are the main points to remember:

- Bedtime and Naptime Routines

  - Be as consistent as possible. If you read your child a story as part of your routine before sleep training, continue to do so.

  - Place him down groggy whenever possible. It's okay if he falls asleep with the bottle, just be sure not to rock him to sleep.

- o If he stands up *and* cries, place him back down, tuck him in, and leave.

- o Use "doorway tricks" if it helps with the transition. For example, we left the bedroom door about a quarter of the way open until he was asleep for the first week... and still sometimes do today!

- o If he keeps waking up and you're at your wit's end, try sitting in the dark room after you put him back down. Just don't pick him up unless you think something's wrong.

- o Determine an appropriate wake-up time beforehand, such as 6:30 a.m. If your toddler wakes up before then, treat it as a midnight waking.

- Midnight Wakings
  - o Do *not* pick him up and rock him back to sleep, feed him, etc.

  - o Lay him back down and tuck him in. Make sure he has his pacifier and lovey, if he uses either of those things. Rub his back a few times and make shushing noises, if he likes them. Sometimes, gently rubbing the top of his head can help to soothe him. Back away and leave the room.

- ○ If he stands up *and* cries, lay him back down, tuck him in, and leave again.

- ○ Here again, tricks like sitting nearby in the room or leaving the door halfway open can help.

- Naps

  - ○ Follow the bedtime procedure.

  - ○ However, recognize that not all naps will be consistent in duration. If he's showing signs of being alert and rested, such as babbling or playing, then nap time should probably be over.

Obviously, pick up your toddler if he sounds hurt. If you smell a poopy diaper, change him and put him back to sleep.

Above all, be consistent... but not dogmatic. Adapt to special situations, such as sickness or painful teething. Don't feel bad if you have to resort to a drive in the car once or twice. If your toddler is freaking out and it's abundantly clear that extreme measures are needed, then go ahead and take him for a drive. Using this tactic very sparingly should not hamper sleep training. Again, use this *only* as a last resort.

Your toddler should learn how to sleep within three or four weeks. If it takes longer, consult your pediatrician.

Get Started

If this method makes sense to you as the right balance between Cry It Out and No Tears, then commit now to making the change. Talk to your partner and make sure you're both on the same page with how you put your toddler to bed, how you respond to midnight wakings, and what time is an acceptable wake-up time.

If you or your partner works a traditional Monday through Friday schedule, you may find it less stressful to start training on a Friday night. That way, you won't be as tempted to give up if it takes an hour — or two! — to put your child to bed the first few nights.

Support

I'd love to hear your success stories, learn about your challenges, and answer any questions you have. Please stop by our website at HelpMyToddlerSleep.com to join the discussion.

Also, visit HelpMyToddlerSleep.com/ Resources to check out the following resources:

- Sample bedtime routine (formatted for printing)

- A printable chart to track sleep training progress

summer of 1780 and the French arrival that we mentioned above. Despite all their worries and exhaustion, both Woodhull and Townsend were still fully committed to the Patriot cause, and they carried their weight on. The ring managed to pick up on some important British maneuvers. They eventually learned that the British were fully aware of the incoming French fleet that was supposed to move on Rhode Island. To that effect, the Brits began moving their own naval forces there to meet the French in combat.

Acting on this information, Washington was able to take action and prevent what could have been a major blow to his French allies. The French Major General Marquis de Lafayette was bringing in some 6,000 troops, aiming to land them at Newport. The Continental Army didn't even have to fight the British to prevent this ambush. Washington simply put his spies to work yet again, instructing them to spread misinformation and create a ruse, making the British think that there was an imminent attack by the Continental Army in New York. This trick worked very well, and a bulk of the British naval forces had to be directed back and instructed to abandon their move to Rhode Island.

This was a major win for the Culper Ring and the Patriot cause as a whole, but Washington would soon run into yet another challenge. This was the defection of Benedict Arnold to the British side, after which he tried to expose as many American spies as he could, leading to a lot of problems for some, including Mulligan.

It was the Culper Ring that first discovered secretive, treacherous communication between Benedict Arnold and John Andre. Andre was the chief of intelligence under the command of British General Henry Clinton in New York. The correspondence between Andre and Arnold concerned the eventual surrender of the American positions at West Point over to the British. This wasn't blackmail or a result of coercion, as Arnold was fully willing to turn the position over to the Brits and defect. In another great accomplishment of the Culper Ring, this plot was foiled, and Andre was eventually captured and hung by the rebels for espionage.

In light of the arrests that occurred following Benedict Arnold's defection, Tallmadge informed Washington in the autumn of 1780 that the Culper network wasn't in jeopardy as Arnold didn't have the information needed to hunt down the main ringleaders. Nonetheless, Woodhull, Townsend, and others were forced to keep a low profile for a while thereafter.

All in all, even the most simplified list of the accomplishments of the Culper Ring and American revolutionary spies, in general, is quite impressive. They helped the French arrive safely, they helped them ambush the British, they kept tabs on British activity, they uncovered treason and plots within American ranks, they prevented the elimination of the Revolution's leader and future first President of the United States.

The accomplishments of the Culper Ring are thus immense and have altered the lives of many folks, not to mention the course of important historical events. It doesn't take a whole lot of thinking to realize how different things could have been if Washington was killed or if certain French reinforcements were decimated at sea. The Culper Ring was formed to keep the Revolution's war machine running smoothly from behind the curtains, and that's exactly what they did.

CHAPTER VI:

~

Interesting Facts

In time, we might get to learn even more new things about the Culper Ring and its exploits. The thing with intelligence networks is that the top-secret nature of their work ensures that a lot of things are buried deep under mounds of silence and deliberate misinformation alike. Even when information gets declassified a long time after the events, it still might take some time for certain dots to be connected, and some things might stay buried forever. Now that you know the main story of how things transpired during those turbulent times, we will also take a look at some other interesting facts about the spy ring, some of which are less well-known than others.

NOTES AND REFERENCES

1. Henderson, J. M. T., France, K. G., Owens, J. L., Blampied, N. M. (2008). Sleeping Through the Night: The Consolidation of Self-regulated Sleep Across the First Year of Life. *Pediatrics, 126*(5), 1081-1087. [URL: http://pediatrics.aappublications.org/content/pediatrics/early/2010/10/25/peds.2010-0976.full.pdf]

2. Guthrie, A. (1997). Separation Anxiety: An Overview. *American Academy of Pediatric Dentistry, 19*(7), 486-489. [URL: http://www.aapd.org/assets/1/25/guthrie-19-08.pdf]

3. Jacobson, J. L., Wille, D. E. (1984). Influence of Attachment and Separation Experience on Separation Distress at 18 months. *Developmental Psychology, 20*(3), 477-484. [URL: http://opensample.info/influence-of-attachment-and-separation-experience-on-separation-distress-at-18-months]

4. Vaughan, C., Dement, W. (1999). The Promise of Sleep. New York: Random House.

5. Iglowstein, I., Jenni, O. G., Molinari, L., Largo, R. H. (2003). Sleep Duration from

Infancy to Adolescence: Reference Values and Generational Trends. *Pediatrics, 111*(2), 302-307. [URL: http://www.ncbi.nlm.nih.gov/pubmed/12563055]

6. Gottlieb, D. J., O'Connor, G T., Wilk, J. B. (2007). Genome-wide Association of Sleep and Circadian Phenotypes. *BMC Medical Genetics, 8*(Supplement 1), S9-S16. [URL: http://www.ncbi.nlm.nih.gov/pubmed/17903308]

7. Ottaviano, S., Giannotti, F., Cortesi, F., Bruni, O., Ottaviano, C. (1996). Sleep Characteristics in Healthy Children from Birth to 6 Years of Age in the Urban Area of Rome. *Sleep, 19*(1), 1-3. [URL: http://www.ncbi.nlm.nih.gov/pubmed/8650456]

8. Lui, X., Lui, L., Wang, R. (2003). Bed Sharing, Sleep Habits, and Sleep Problems Among Chinese School-Aged Children. *Sleep, 26*(7), 839-844. [URL: http://www.ncbi.nlm.nih.gov/pubmed/14655917]

9. Super, C. M., Harkness, S., Van Tijen, N. (1996). Parents' Cultural Belief Systems: Their Origins, Expressions, and Consequences. New York: Guilford Press.

10. Narvaez, D. "Dangers of 'Crying It Out." *Psychology Today*. Psychology Today, 11 December 2011. Web (https://www.psychologytoday.com/blog/moral-landscapes/201112/dangers-crying-it-out). 23 September 2016 Accessed.

11. Sears, W., Sears, M. "Let Baby Cry It Out." *Ask Dr. Sears*. AskDrSears.com, 29 August 2013. Web (http://www.askdrsears.com/topics/health-concerns/fussy-baby/letting-baby-cry-it-out-yes-no). 23 September 2016 Accessed.

12. Price, A. M. H., Wake, M., Ukoumunne, O. C., Hiscock, H. (2012) Five-Year Follow-up of Harms and Benefits of Behavioral Infant Sleep Intervention: Randomized Trial. *Pediatrics, 130*(4), 2011-3467. [URL: http://www.ncbi.nlm.nih.gov/pubmed/22966034]

About the Author

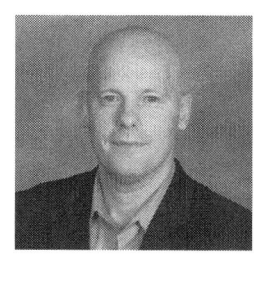

Paul is married to Kristee, the love of his life. They met in Roseville, MN and spent their first five years together in St. Paul. In 2015, they fled the frigid Minnesota winters and relocated to the Gulf Coast in Florida. They have two boys, one in preschool and one still in diapers.

Paul owns a technology consulting company and is an occasional contributor to parenting blogs. This is his first book.